THE HEALTHY LOWER BACK

Laying the Foundation Through
— *Proper Lifting, Sitting, and Exercise* —

By

DENNIS ZACHARKOW, R.P.T.

Department of Physical Medicine and Rehabilitation
Mayo Clinic
Rochester, Minnesota

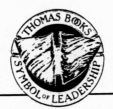

CHARLES C THOMAS • PUBLISHER
Springfield • Illinois • U.S.A.

Published and Distributed Throughout the World by

CHARLES C THOMAS • PUBLISHER
2600 South First Street
Springfield, Illinois 62717

© *1984 by* CHARLES C THOMAS • PUBLISHER

ISBN 0-398-04984-X

Library of Congress Catalog Card Number: 83-24295

With THOMAS BOOKS *careful attention is given to all details of manufacturing and design. It is the Publisher's desire to present books that are satisfactory as to their physical qualities and artistic possibilities and appropriate for their particular use.* THOMAS BOOKS *will be true to those laws of quality that assure a good name and good will.*

Printed in the United States of America
Q-R-3

Library of Congress Cataloging in Publication Data

Zacharkow, Dennis
  The healthy lower back.

  Bibliography: p.
  Includes index.
    1. Back—Care and hygiene. 2. Exercise. 3. Backache—Prevention.
I. Title. [DNLM: 1. Back—Popular works.
2. Gymnastics. WE 720 Z16h]
RD768.Z33   1984   617 '.56052   83-2495
ISBN 0-398-04984-X

To
Robert Collier

PREFACE

Taking responsibility for the proper care of one's lower back when young is the best assurance for keeping one's lower back healthy throughout life. The younger a person is, the easier it will be to learn the proper muscular control of the lower back, along with the proper way to lift, sit, and exercise. The older one gets, the more ingrained improper techniques and incorrect movement patterns will be.[12] These habits will then be extremely difficult to correct.

Therefore, this book is intended to be used primarily by physical education and health teachers from the elementary school to the university level. Other professionals involved in teaching preventive back care to the public, physical therapists, occupational therapists, nurses, physicians, and occupational health and safety consultants, will also benefit from the principles discussed in this book.

This book's exercise program is designed to train people specifically for the lifting and sitting in their daily activities. Once mastered, all the recommended exercises can be done independently.

Even though the exercise program is intended for adolescents and young adults with healthy backs, a physician should still be consulted before attempting any of the exercises discussed in this book. These exercises should not be done by individuals with acute back pain or chronic back problems, advanced degenerative changes or structural defects of the spine, knee problems, high blood pressure, or other cardiorespiratory problems.

This book's exercise program is not intended as a total exercise program to correct all postural faults and strengthen all muscle groups, but only to improve one's lifting and sitting posture.

The technical terminology pertaining to the lower back has been minimized so that this book will be readable for individuals seeking advice on preventive back care from various health professionals. For those individuals interested in more detailed technical reading, superior numbers are used throughout the text to refer to the references listed in the bibliography.

The views expressed in this book are solely those of the author, and not of the Mayo Clinic.

ACKNOWLEDGMENTS

Many thanks to the following individuals:

Robert Collier, John H. Maxwell, and David Leitch for their influence on the author's weight training and exercise philosophy.

Lee Huber and Luke Klaja, R.P.T., for sharing their knowledge on Olympic weight lifting techniques.

Robert H. Graebe and Robert L. Keith for their friendship.

Rich Shields, R.P.T., Ken Lennington, R.P.T., Julie Bass, O.T.R., Tom McCoy, D.O., and Roger Klauer, M.D., for reviewing the manuscript.

David Franzen for his work on the line illustrations.

Lana Kelsey for typing the manuscript.

CONTENTS

THE HEALTHY LOWER BACK

Chapter 1

INTRODUCTION

It has been estimated that 80 percent of all individuals, at one time or another, will be afflicted with low back pain.[75] During the present decade, on a worldwide scale, about two billion people will seek treatment for low back pain.[75]

Low back pain is the most common cause of "occupational and domestic disability in industrialized societies."[105] The cost for the treatment and compensation of low back pain in the United States is approximately $14 billion each year.[99]

Although much is still unknown regarding the causes of low back pain, mechanical factors are often involved either primarily or secondarily in many low back problems.[13,14,27,33,41,54,74,75,78,87,92]

It is the premise of this book that low back problems involving mechanical stress frequently develop from poor posture, poor lifting techniques, and improper exercises learned in childhood and adolescence and continued as adults.

All of these potentially harmful habits may result in excessive wear and tear of the discs, the shock absorbing pads located between the bones (vertebrae) of the spinal column (Fig. 1). Disc problems usually develop in the lower back (lumbar spine). This is the area of the back subject to the greatest mechanical stress. The disc has been implicated as a major cause of low back pain.[75]

As prolonged wear and tear on the healthy lumbar spine result in disc degeneration, abnormal stresses may then develop in the posterior joints (facet joints) located between the vertebrae (Fig. 1), resulting in another potential site for low back pain.[75]

In addition, poor posture, poor lifting techniques, and improper exercises learned in childhood and adolescence can also make one more susceptible to another possible source of low back pain—acute back sprains and strains involving the posterior ligaments and muscles of the lower back.[1,23,78,100]

3

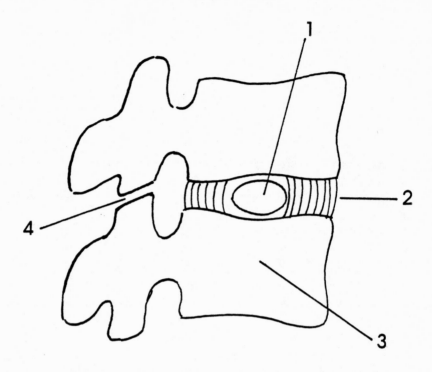

Figure 1. (1) Nucleus pulposus, the gelatinous central region of the disc. (2) Annulus fibrosus, the fibrous wall of the disc. (3) Vertebra (4) Facet joint.

In order for man to stand upright with straight knees, a slight curve or arch evolved in the lower back, referred to as the normal lumbar lordosis (Fig. 2).[8] This is the normal physiological position for the lower back when one stands upright.[71] Standing with the knees straight and the normal lumbar lordosis requires less muscle activity than standing with the knees slightly bent and a flat lower back (Fig. 3).[10]

Along with the other flexible curves of the human spine (Fig. 4), this normal lumbar lordosis results in the spine being ten times stronger than if it were perfectly straight.[43] Several authors feel that more back problems result from the loss of this normal lumbar lordosis into a straight or flat back posture.[16,27,50,63,102]

Improper lifting technique and poor sitting posture are considered to be two of the major predisposing factors to low back

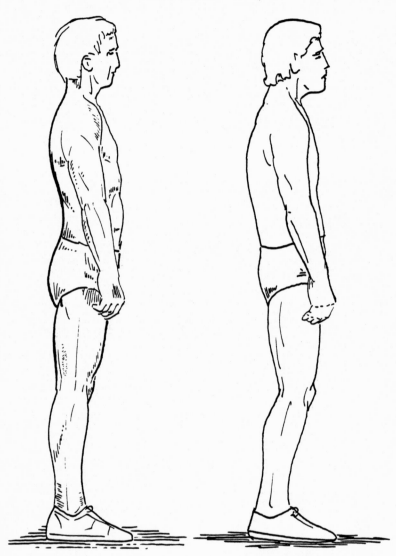

Figure 2. Normal lumbar lordosis in upright standing.

Figure 3. Flat lower back, as opposed to the normal lumbar lordosis in upright standing.

pain.[16, 44, 54, 63–65, 73] The frequency of lifting heavy objects and sitting is extremely high in our society compared to our ancestors.[18]

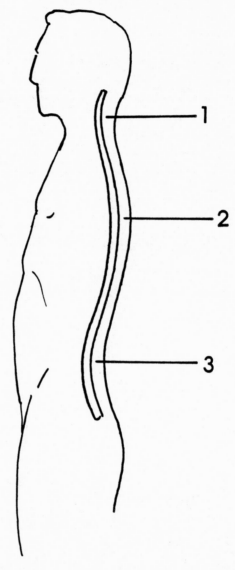

Figure 4. The three normal flexible curves of the spine: (1) Cervical curve. (2) Thoracic curve. (3) Lumbar curve.

However, the normal protective curve of the lower back that evolved for erect upright stance and locomotion is easily lost when lifting and sitting. Proper lifting and sitting postures maintaining this curve do not come naturally, but are acquired skills that must be learned and practiced.[12]

Unfortunately, the vast majority of the population are unable to obtain the correct lifting technique due to a lack of proper flexibility, muscle weakness, or a lack of skill and coordination specific to lifting. Many people are unaware of how to properly contract the lower back muscles when lifting. Lifelong habits of exercising in flexion patterns such as toe touches with the knees straight and full sit-ups that eliminate and reverse the normal lumbar lordosis have also contributed to ingraining poor lifting techniques in many people.

As a result of these deficits and habits, one will be constantly predisposed to low back injury. The lower to the ground one has to lift from, the more difficult maintaining proper lifting technique will be. (Seventy-eight percent of industrial back injuries from lifting are due to lifting from below 31 inches, or knuckle height.)[87]

Similarly, due to a lack of necessary flexibility for proper sitting posture, and from prolonged sitting in poorly designed chairs in which it is difficult to maintain the normal lumbar lordosis, one will be constantly predisposed to low back stress.

This book's exercise program is designed to train people specifically for the lifting involved in their daily activities. The same exercises will also assure that one has the necessary flexibility and strength to sit properly.

In the final chapter, several popular exercises performed in physical education classes, and physical fitness and weight training programs, will be discussed regarding their potential harm to the lower back.

CHAPTER 2

LIFTING

The most harmful position for stressing the discs, ligaments, and muscles of the lower back is forward bending (flexion).[1,2,23,38,52,78] This can either be pure forward bending, or forward bending combined with side bending (lateral flexion), or twisting (rotation) (Figs. 5–7).[1,28,38,51,52] Lateral flexion and rotation occur as parts of a combined movement, rather than as totally separate, isolated movements.[68,70]

These flexed postures are the most dangerous because they will result in maximum stretching of the posterior fibrous wall (annulus fibrosus) of the disc, the disc's weakest area (Fig. 8).[39,66,72,86] This stretching is caused by the posterior movement of the disc's gelatinous central region (nucleus pulposus) when the lower back is in flexion.[43,86]

The opposite position from flexion of the lower back is called extension (backward bending) (Fig. 9). The safest position for the lower back when lifting is to maintain a slightly extended or arched position, referred to as a lordotic lifting posture. With this lifting posture, the lower back muscles will have the greatest mechanical advantage.[23,95]

Compared to flexion, keeping the lower back slightly arched will decrease the stress on the posterior part of the disc.[86] The pressure within the disc will also be less compared to flexion.[77] With a slightly arched position, some of the weight bearing will be taken off the discs and distributed to the facet joints.[48,59,60,62] This is the most stable position for the lumbar spine, since the facet joints are *locked,* and minimal motion is possible between the individual vertebrae.[29,53] The discs will therefore be protected from any twisting forces when lifting. In a flexed position, with the facet joints *unlocked* (see Fig. 8), there is a greater potential for a twisting motion to occur and damage the discs.[42]

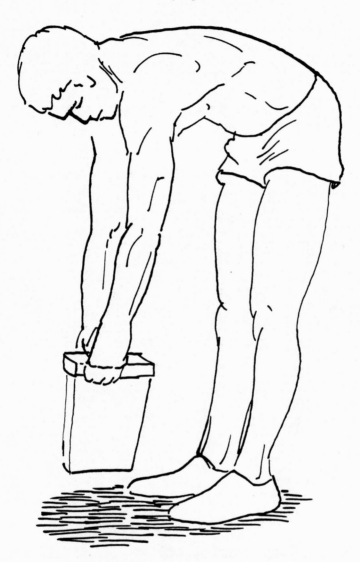

Figure 5. Lifting with the lower back in flexion.

REASONS FOR IMPROPER LIFTING POSTURE

Most people have at one time heard the expression, "Lift with your legs and not your back." However, even if this statement is

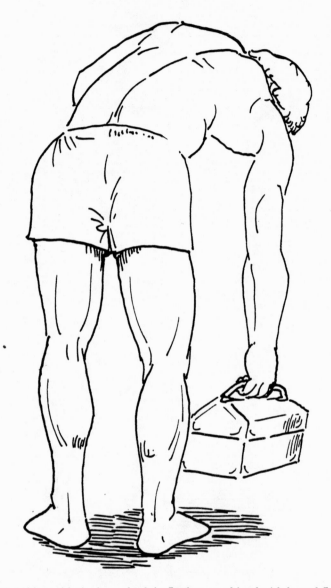

Figure 6. Lifting with the lower back in flexion, combined with lateral flexion.

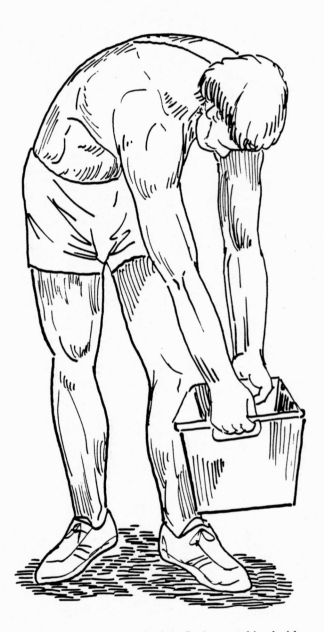

Figure 7. Lifting with the lower back in flexion, combined with rotation.

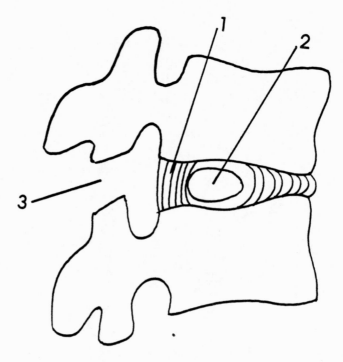

Figure 8. Maximum stretching of the posterior annulus fibrosus (1) in flexion, due to the posterior movement of the nucleus pulposus (2). Note the unlocked position of the facet joint (3).

understood, the vast majority of the population will still not be able to squat down and lift properly, with a slight arch in the lower back.

The main reasons for improper lifting posture are as follows.

Tight Calf Muscles

An individual with tight calf muscles will be forced to raise his heels off the floor and balance on his toes as he squats down to a near parallel position while maintaining a slight arch in his lower back (Fig. 10). Since it is difficult to balance when squatting on one's toes, and even more difficult to lift an object in this position, the individual will usually flex his lower back and let his heels touch the floor (Fig. 11). The individual will then have better balance but will be in greater danger of injuring his lower back.

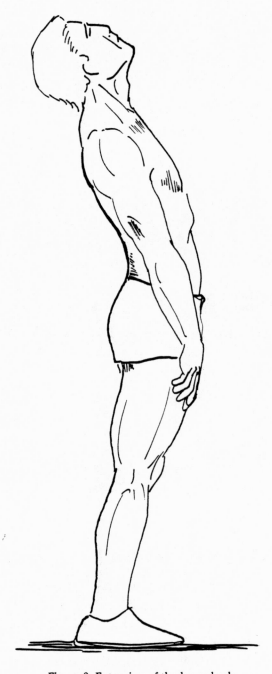

Figure 9. Extension of the lower back.

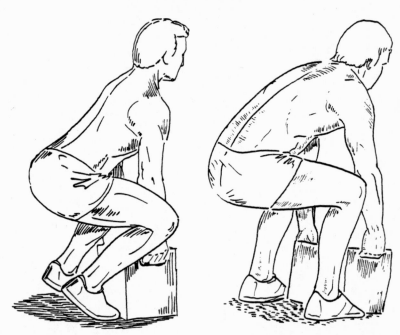

Figure 10. Squatting up on the toes due to   Figure 11. Squatting with the
tight calf muscles.   heels on the floor,* but the
                                                    lower back in flexion.

The key is to get the calf muscles as loose as possible (*see* leg
stretching exercise number one in Chapter 4). However, even
without calf muscle tightness, the majority of individuals will still
not have sufficient ankle mobility to easily keep their heels on the
floor when squatting down to a near parallel position with a slight
arch in the lower back and the body weight over or just behind the
balls of the feet. This is why the proper heel height in shoes to
improve one's balance is very important for people doing a lot of
lifting from low heights, such as in industrial settings, household
jobs, or weight lifting exercise programs.

For most individuals, a wide heel with a ½ to 1 inch (1.3
to 2.5 cm) heel to sole height difference on shoes with good
ankle support will improve one's balance and allow the normal lumbar lordosis of the erect standing posture to be func-
tional for lifting from low heights. Very low heeled shoes, such
as running shoes, should only be worn in lifting situations

by individuals with excellent ankle flexibility.

Negative heel shoes, which have a higher sole height than heel height, should not be worn when one is lifting. The same applies to going barefoot. In these instances, one will either lift in the unstable position of balancing on one's toes or else improve one's balance by having the entire foot make contact with the floor, but with a flexed back.

Tight Hamstrings

When the hamstrings are tight, the range of pure hip flexion without spinal flexion will be limited. Therefore, as one squats down to a position where the thighs are near parallel to the floor, the lower back will also flex due to the hamstrings' pull on the pelvis (Fig. 12). Leg stretching exercise number two in Chapter 4 is very important to prevent hamstring tightness.

Tight Gluteus Maximus

Tightness in this muscle group will have the same effect as tight hamstrings when one squats down to a near parallel position (*see* Fig. 12). Leg stretching exercise number three, Chapter 4, is very important to stretch the gluteus maximus muscle and increase the range of pure hip flexion.

Lack of Mobility in Back Extension

Some individuals will be unable to obtain a lordosis when lifting because they are unable to extend their backs sufficiently.[63] This is due to keeping the lower back flexed day after day through poor sitting and standing postures, and flexion exercise programs. As a result, these individuals never fully extend their lower backs. The standing back extension exercise in Chapter 4 is important to assure sufficient mobility in extension.

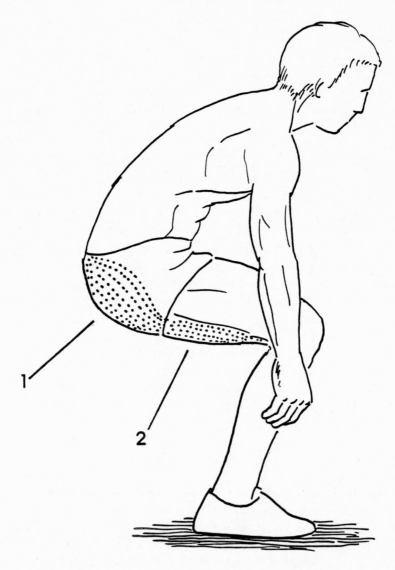

Figure 12. When squatting, tight hamstring (2) and gluteus maximus (1) muscles will force the lower back to flex due to their pull on the pelvis.

Muscle Weakness

The most important muscles to be strengthened for proper lifting technique are the lumbar erector spinae (lower back muscles), quadriceps, gluteus maximus, hamstrings, gastrocnemius, and soleus (Fig. 13). These muscles must be strengthened specific to the movement and function desired.[34,85] This is different from just exercising isolated muscle groups. For example, there will be a lack of carry-over to proper lifting technique if one just strengthens the quadriceps muscles by doing resistive knee extension exercises (Fig. 14).

A multiple joint movement, such as the parallel squat (resistive exercise number one, Chap. 4), will strengthen all the critical muscle groups in the specific movement desired (Fig. 15). With the proper squat technique, the lower back muscles will be strengthened as stabilizers of the lumbar spine, their most important function for protecting against back injuries.

Incoordination With Lifting Technique

It takes much practice to develop the skill, coordination, and balance to lift properly. This includes learning how to properly contract the lower back muscles when lifting. The parallel squat is an excellent exercise to develop these components of proper lifting technique.

Weak Upper Back

With a weak upper back, the individual will tend to lift with the upper back rounded and shoulders forward. This posture will also tend to flex the lower back when lifting (Fig. 16). Resistive exercise number two, Chapter 4, is important to strengthen the upper back.

Tight Clothing

Certain clothing, such as tight-fitting jeans, will not allow enough free motion at the hips to squat properly. One will therefore be forced to flex the lower back when lifting objects from low heights.

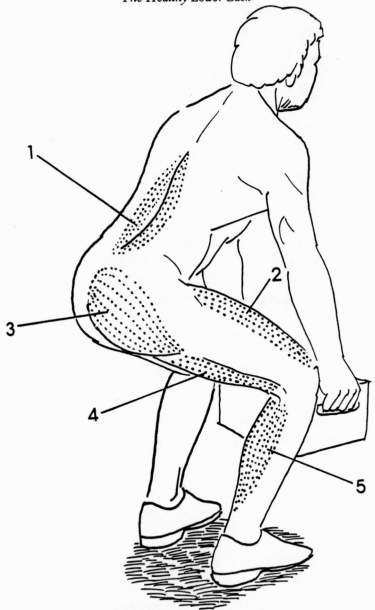

Figure 13. Important muscles to be strengthened for proper lifting technique: (1) Erector spinae (back extensors). (2) Quadriceps (knee extensors). (3) Gluteus maximus (hip extensor). (4) Hamstrings (hip extensors). (5) Calf muscles—gastrocnemius and soleus (ankle extensors).

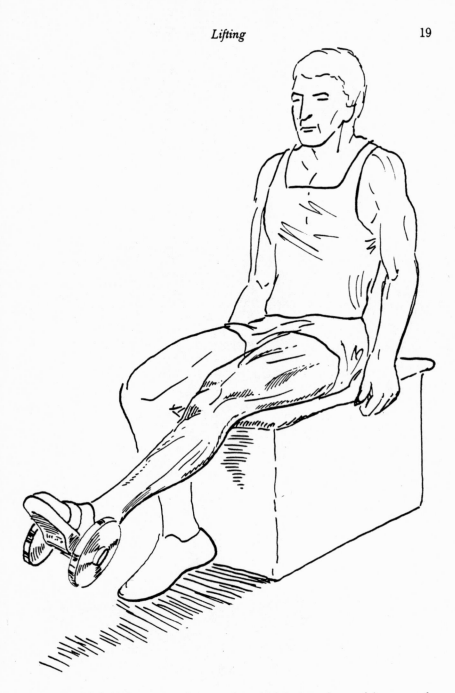

Figure 14. Resistive knee extension exercise, which isolates the quadriceps muscle group.

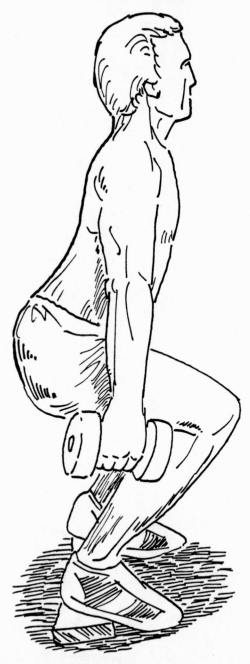

Figure 15. Parallel squat, a multiple joint movement important for proper lifting technique.

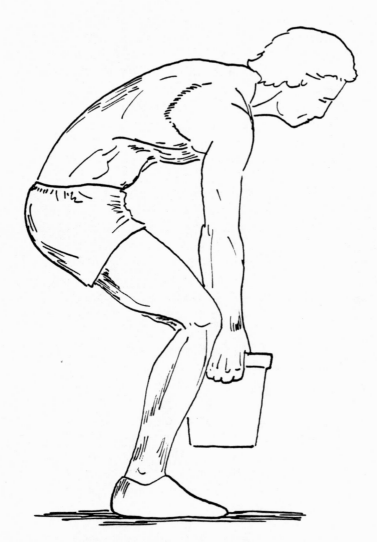

Figure 16. Lifting with a weak upper back.

CORRECT LIFTING TECHNIQUE

1. To properly protect the discs and ligaments, the lower back muscles must be consciously contracted at the start of the lift.[60, 81]

This is important to practice, since many individuals are unaware of the feeling of tightening their lower back muscles and keeping them contracted throughout the lift. This tightening should eventually become second nature and should be done regardless of how light the object being lifted is. In addition, the lower back muscles should also be contracted when pushing and pulling objects. (Interestingly, with tasks requiring increased activity from the lumbar erector spinae muscles, individuals with chronic low back pain show less activation of these muscles than individuals without back pain.)[15]

2. It is extremely important to keep the object being lifted as close to the body as possible (Fig. 17).[6] An object being lifted from in front of the feet should always be brought in closer to the body as it is raised off the floor.

3. Lifting should always be done slowly, as a slow lift from the floor results in less stress on the back compared to a fast lift.[17,19] Without adequate practice, unskilled individuals often raise their hips too fast when lifting, and therefore end up flexing their lower back (Fig. 18).[20]

4. Unskilled individuals often keep their neck flexed instead of slightly extended when lifting, which then causes the entire spine to flex.[91] One should think of "looking up" at the start of a heavy lift from the floor to assure good spinal posture.

5. When lowering a weight or object to the ground, one must keep the lower back muscles contracted, and the lumbar spine in a slightly arched position. Even after good lifting technique from the floor, many individuals often forget this and end up relaxing their back muscles and flexing their lumbar spine when lowering an object to the floor.

6. A twisting motion should never be done when lifting an object. At the completion of a lift, one should rotate the feet while moving an object to the side, rather than keeping the feet immobile and twisting the trunk only (Fig. 19).

7. When lifting with a slight arch in the lower back, the trunk will not be perfectly vertical. If one is able to straddle the object that is being lifted, the trunk will usually be inclined approximately 20 to 40 degrees from vertical (Fig. 20). With objects being

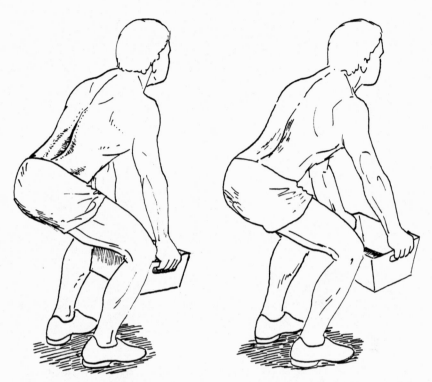

Figure 17. The object being lifted should be kept as close to the body as possible. a. Correct. b. Incorrect.

lifted from in front of the feet, this angle may be from 30 to 70 degrees (Fig. 21).

The trunk angle in a certain lifting situation will vary between individuals, depending on one's height and body proportions. The trunk angle will also vary for the same individual depending on how low the object being lifted is from the ground. Objects being lifted from in front of the feet and very close to the ground will require the greatest trunk angle from vertical.

8. At the start of the lift, the body weight should be over or just behind the balls of the feet, not over the heels. Having the body weight over or just behind the balls of the feet will reduce the stress on the lower back, since the individual's lumbar spine will be closer to the object being lifted (Fig. 22).

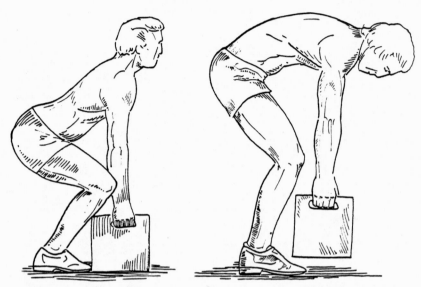

Figure 18. Raising the hips too fast at the start of a lift. a. Correct starting position. b. Incorrect. The hips raise too fast.

COMPARISON OF DIFFERENT LIFTING POSTURES

The proper lordotic lifting technique is illustrated in Figure 23. This technique should be compared to the other frequently performed lifting postures described later.

Full Spinal Flexion

Lifting with the back in extreme flexion (Fig. 24) is an easy habit to develop. Individuals with tight hamstrings, gluteus maximus, and calf muscles, and weak leg muscles overall will often lift from this position. This lifting posture potentially can be very dangerous, because in the fully flexed position the back muscles are relaxed, and all the stress is on the posterior aspect of the discs and posterior ligaments of the back.[26,32,97,103]

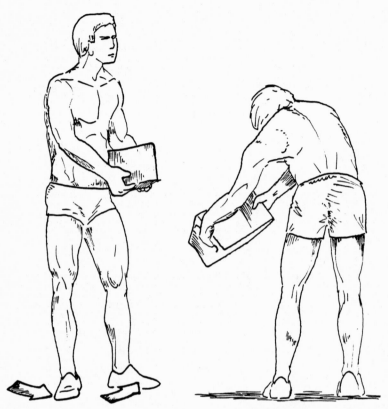

Figure 19. a. Proper rotation of the feet when moving an object to the side at the completion of a lift. b. Incorrect. The feet are kept immobile and only the trunk rotates.

Slight Spinal Flexion

Lifting in a position of slight spinal flexion is frequently advocated as the proper lifting technique. The individual is taught to keep his pelvis upwardly rotated by tightening his abdominal muscles as he squats down to lift an object.

With this lifting posture, the individual's lower back muscles will be fairly relaxed at the start of the lift, and his body weight will be over his heels.[11] The individual's lumbar spine in this

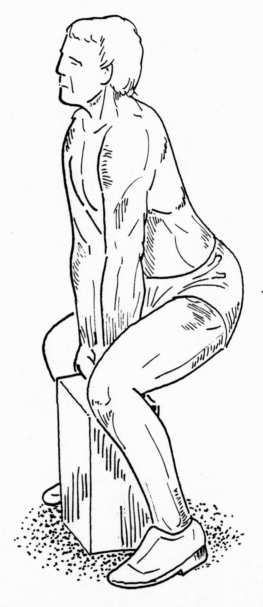

Figure 20. Trunk angle when lifting a low object that can be straddled.

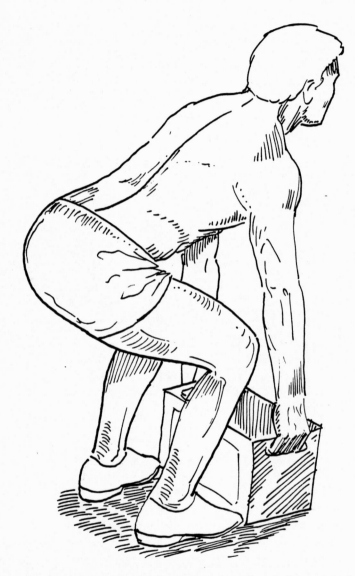

Figure 21. Trunk angle when lifting a low object from in front of the feet.

flexed posture will be farther away from the object being lifted, compared to a slightly arched lifting posture, resulting in greater stress on the lower back (Fig. 25).

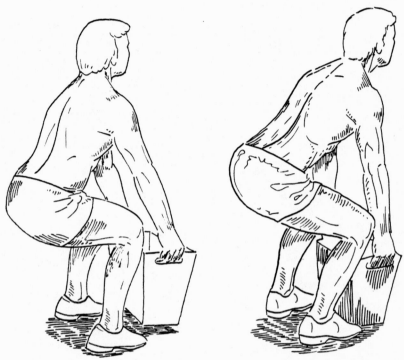

Figure 22. a. Incorrect. At the start of the lift, the body weight is over the heels. b. Correct. At the start of the lift, the body weight is over or just behind the balls of the feet.

Vertical Trunk and Straight Back

Squatting down to lift while keeping the trunk vertical and the back straight will be a very unstable lifting posture, since the individual will have to balance up on his toes (Fig. 26). Lifting illustrations that show an individual's trunk perfectly upright with the feet flat on the floor are inaccurate, since this posture is extremely difficult to assume and maintain at the start of a lift.

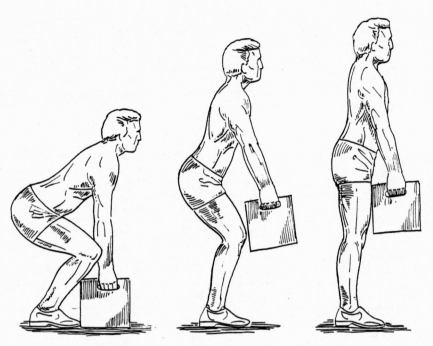

Figure 23. Sequence of proper lifting technique.

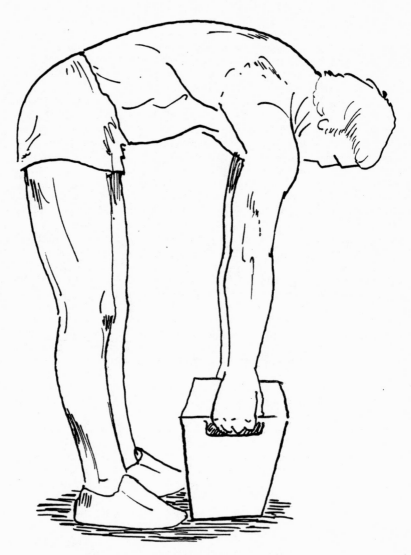

Figure 24. Lifting with the lower back in extreme flexion.

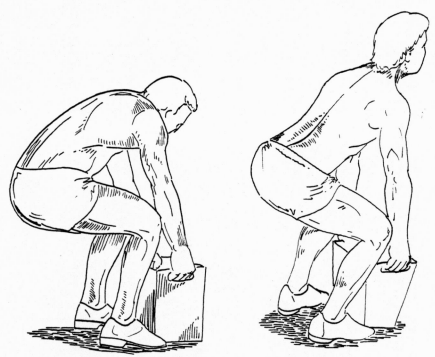

Figure 25. a. Lifting with the lower back in slight flexion and the body weight over the heels. b. Correct lordotic lifting posture.

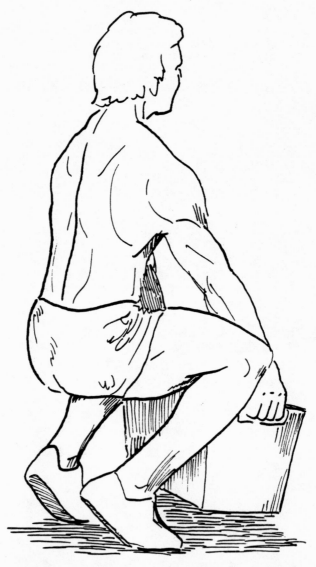

Figure 26. Balancing up on the toes with a vertical trunk and straight back, an unstable lifting posture.

Chapter 3

IMPORTANCE OF ABDOMINAL MUSCLES

Proper strengthening of the abdominal muscles is critical due to their importance in protecting the lower back from injury when lifting. This is because the increase in pressure within the abdominal cavity (intra-abdominal pressure) that occurs when a person lifts a heavy object from the floor can relieve some of the excessive load on the lumbar vertebrae and discs.[9,24,25]

Sit-up exercises primarily strengthen the rectus abdominis muscle group, with a greater intensity of contraction from the upper rectus compared to the lower rectus (Fig. 27).[61,83] The rectus muscles, however, contract minimally or not at all when lifting or straining, as their primary function is to flex the trunk.[9,31,79,88] With the great increase in disc pressure and the extreme lumbar spinal flexion that occur with full sit-ups, disc degeneration may be accelerated.[37,101]

The basic pattern of abdominal muscle activity used in lifting to increase the intra-abdominal pressure is the exact opposite of the sit-up movement.[31,79] It consists of an isometric abdominal contraction—the muscles contract without causing any trunk movement.

This abdominal muscle contraction is most likely a reflex that is related to the magnitude of contraction of the erector spinae muscles.[24,56-58] The greater the contraction of the erector spinae muscles, the greater the contraction of the abdominal muscles will be to reduce the stress on the spine.

Parts of the oblique abdominal muscles and the transversus abdominal muscle (Figs. 27 and 28) are probably involved in this isometric abdominal muscle contraction.[9,82] These muscles will help increase the intra-abdominal pressure without flexing the lumbar spine.

The transversus abdominal muscle and lower anterior internal

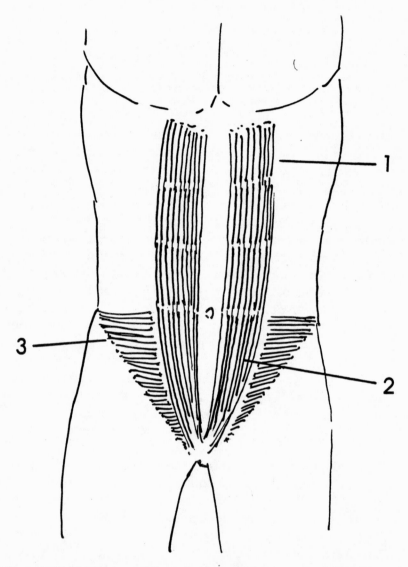

Figure 27. (1) Upper rectus abdominis muscle. (2) Lower rectus abdominis muscle. (3) Lower anterior internal oblique abdominal muscle.

oblique abdominal muscle will not flex the lumbar spine because the muscle fibers run in a horizontal direction. In addition, the

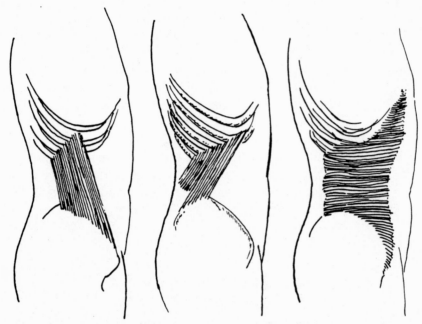

Figure 28. a. Lateral (posterior) fibers of the external oblique abdominal muscle. b. Lateral (posterior) fibers of the internal oblique abdominal muscle. c. Transversus abdominal muscle.

lower anterior internal oblique abdominal muscle and the lower portion of the transversus muscle will support the organs within the abdominal cavity by preventing any bulging of the lower abdominal wall.[79]

The most lateral (posterior) muscle fibers of the external and internal obliques will contribute minimally to lumbar spinal flexion, since they do not have an anterior location on the abdominal wall.[82] These fibers will also help stabilize the trunk laterally when lifting.

At the beginning of a heavy lift, when the individual keeps a slight arch in the lower back and takes a deep breath, the abdominal muscles will be slightly stretched, and therefore be in a more advantageous position to develop tension for their isometric contraction.[89] By the individual focusing on contracting the lower back muscles when lifting, the abdominal muscles will contract reflexly as needed to reduce the stress on the spine.

The stronger the abdominal muscles are in performing an isometric contraction, the more protection one will have for the spine when lifting heavy objects. This abdominal muscle contraction will be particularly important with greater angles of trunk inclination from vertical.[17,24,36]

The exercise that parallels the abdominal muscles' actual function in lifting better than the sit-up is a properly performed isometric leg raise (*see* Fig. 29 and resistive exercise number three, Chapter 4). The isometric leg raise involves a lesser increase in disc pressure than the sit-up and strengthens isometrically all the abdominal muscles important for lifting and stabilizing the pelvis.[31,76,79]

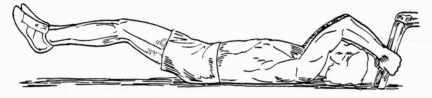

Figure 29. Isometric leg raise.

The isometric leg raise also strengthens the abdominal muscles for their role in maintaining the proper alignment of the pelvis and lumbar spine in the erect standing position. Weakness and overstretching of the lower obliques and transversus muscles will cause the lower abdomen to protrude, with a forward displacement of the pelvis. In order to prevent a forward displacement of the center of gravity, the upper trunk will deviate backwards (Fig. 30). There will also be a rounded posture of the upper back and shoulders.

Although the soft tissue contours of a protruding abdomen and backward deviated upper trunk give the appearance of an excessive lumbar lordosis, the lordosis is usually less than normal with this standing posture.

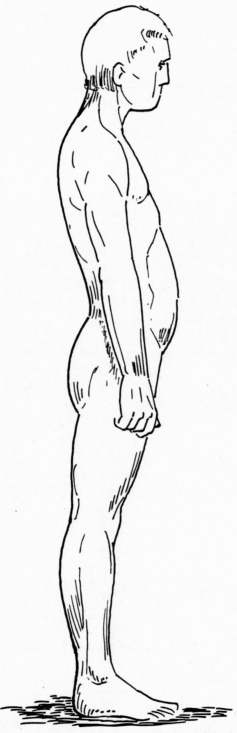

Figure 30. Slouched standing posture due to weakness of the lower obliques and transversus muscles.

Chapter 4

EXERCISE PROGRAM TO IMPROVE LIFTING TECHNIQUE

The rationale behind an exercise program to improve lifting technique is as follows:

A. The leg stretching exercises help to develop the necessary flexibility in the muscle groups that will allow one to lift with the proper lumbar lordosis: the calf muscles, hamstrings, and gluteus maximus.

B. The standing back extension exercise will help achieve or maintain the mobility of the spine necessary for proper lifting technique.

C. The resistive exercises are all related to the lifting movement. The parallel squat strengthens the critical muscles to be used in lifting, specific to their function in lifting. The lower back muscles are strengthened as stabilizers of the spine, their most important function. One also develops the coordination for lifting by practicing this movement.[34, 98]

The shrug exercise, by strengthening and preventing rounding of the upper back, also helps to reinforce proper lifting technique.

The isometric leg raise strengthens the abdominal muscles used in lifting to increase the intra-abdominal pressure.

LEG STRETCHES

Each of the following stretches should be held for one to two minutes.

1. Calf Stretch

Stand arm's length from a wall, keeping one leg in front of the other, with the toes pointed slightly outward. Keep the knee of the front leg bent and the knee of the back leg straight. Slowly bend the elbows and lean into the wall, bending the front knee (Fig. 31). Lean into the wall until a mild stretch is felt in the calf muscles of the back leg. Make sure the heel of the back foot does not raise off the floor during the stretch.

After holding this position for thirty seconds to one minute, change the position of the front leg until it is only slightly ahead of the back leg. Continue the same stretch, only this time allow the back knee to bend (Fig. 32). Allowing the back knee to bend will localize the stretch to the deeper calf muscle (soleus), which does not cross the knee joint. Continue the stretch in this position for another thirty seconds to one minute.

Repeat the same stretch for the opposite leg.

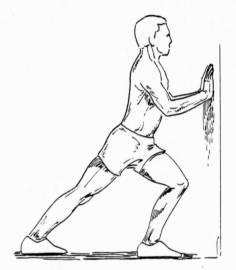 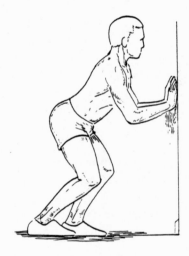

Figure 31. Calf stretch (part one).   Figure 32. Calf stretch (part two).

2. Hamstring Stretch

Lie on the back. Keep one leg firmly against the floor to prevent the lower back from flexing excessively. During the stretch, the lower back should only be flattened against the floor and not flexed any further.

Place a rope around the arch of the foot of the other leg, and with the knee straight (but not forcefully locked), slowly raise the leg upwards until a mild stretch is felt behind the knee (Fig. 33). The eventual goal with this stretch should be to elevate the leg to 85 to 90 degrees, but not any further.[45]

Repeat the same stretch for the opposite leg.

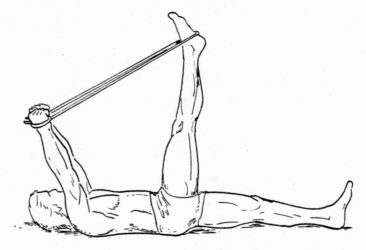

Figure 33. Hamstring stretch.

The advantage of this hamstring stretch over other techniques is that by firmly holding one leg against the floor, one will avoid overstretching the lower back. The stretch will then be better localized to the hamstrings. It is easy to grade one's progress in this stretch by comparing the angle of the stretched leg to the vertical position.

Hamstring tightness is not just limited to the adult population. It is also very common in early adolescence.[46] Around this age, tight hamstrings may possibly lead one to develop poor lifting habits due to the decreased hip mobility.

3. Gluteus Maximus Stretch

Lie on the back. Keep one leg firmly against the floor. For this exercise, do not let the lower back flatten, but maintain a slight arch in the lower back throughout the stretch.

Place both hands just below the other knee, and slowly bring this leg, with the knee bent, toward the chest until a mild stretch is felt in the buttocks region (Fig. 34).

Repeat the same stretch for the opposite leg.

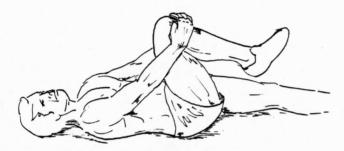

Figure 34. Gluteus maximus stretch.

BACK MOBILITY—STANDING BACK EXTENSION

Without adequate back mobility in extension, it will be impossible to obtain the necessary lordosis for lifting. If one is not used to extending the lumbar spine, this exercise may cause slight discomfort at first.

With hands resting on the front of the thighs, move the hips and abdomen forward. Then, gradually lean backward as far as possible (Fig. 35). The lower back muscles should be relaxed during this exercise. The leaning back is controlled by the gradual lengthening of the abdominal muscles and secondarily by the lengthening of the hip flexor muscles.[47]

Slowly return to the fully upright position. Repeat this exercise for ten repetitions.

RESISTIVE EXERCISES

The following resistive exercises are intended to be done with light weights, with the emphasis on good technique. This program is not meant to be done straining with maximum weights.

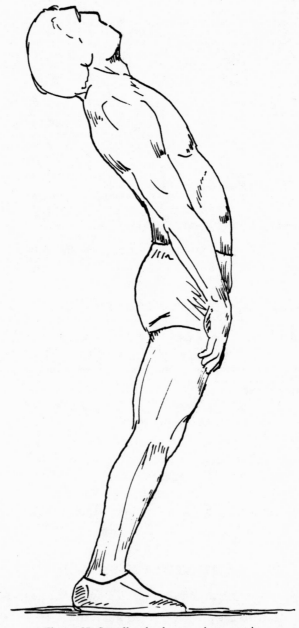

Figure 35. Standing back extension exercise.

With proper instruction and supervision, these exercises can be started around age twelve. (Isometric strength of the trunk muscles has been shown to increase significantly with a strengthening program for prepubescent boys.[96])

Two sets of ten repetitions can be done for each exercise. The first set of ten repetitions should be done without weights. The second set should then be done with a light weight that can be lifted with mild effort for ten repetitions, with good technique. To assure good technique, start the resistive exercises with a one pound (0.5 kg) weight in each hand.

1. Parallel Squat

Holding a dumbell, sandbag, or other weight in each hand, with the feet approximately shoulder width apart and the toes pointed slightly outward, slowly bend the hips and knees until the tops of the thighs are two to three inches above parallel to the floor (Fig. 36). At the start of the squat, keep the head up and tighten the lower back muscles to hold the lumbar spine in an arched position. By exaggerating the arch at the start of the squat, it will be easier to maintain a slight arch at the lowest squat position.

The trunk should not be vertical during the squat but should be inclined slightly forward. Usually, with good technique, the angle of the trunk from vertical will be approximately 15 to 30 degrees. The body weight should be distributed over and behind the balls of the feet, not over the heels during the squat.

At first, you may not be able to squat to near parallel without flattening the lower back. Therefore, stop as soon as you begin to lose the arch in the lower back. Then, keeping your head up, return to the starting position. Inhale before descending into the squat position, and exhale on the way up to the erect position.

It will help to have another person observe your technique, or else use a mirror.

Experiment with a board under your heels, up to approximately two inches (5 cm), to determine how much heel lift is necessary to keep from going up on your toes when squatting. As your calf muscles loosen, the thickness of the board can be reduced.

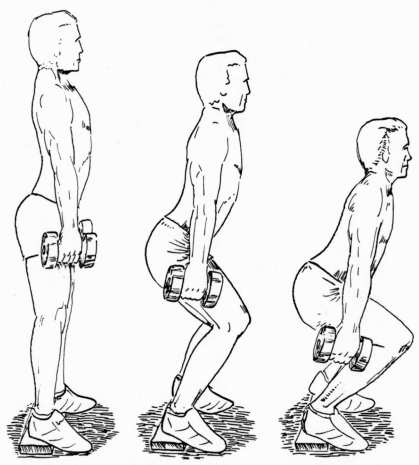

Figure 36. Parallel squat exercise. a. Starting position. b. Middescent. c. Bottom position.

Eventually, you can determine the ideal heel height needed on shoes when doing lifting activities. The ideal heel height will reduce the stress in the calf muscles and improve one's balance when lifting from low heights. Usually, no more than a one-half-to-one-inch (1.3 to 2.5 cm) heel to sole height difference will be needed.

Be careful to do the squat exercise slowly, and do not bounce at the bottom position. Avoid moving the knees together when squatting. Try to keep the knees in the same position throughout the lift.[7] This exercise takes much practice at first in order to develop the necessary balance and coordination.

Proper lifting technique is very similar to this exercise (*see* Chapter 2). When lifting a single object, however, it should be placed in front of the body, not to the side, and as close to the body as possible (Fig. 37). If possible, the object should be placed between, rather than in front of, the legs (Fig. 38).

2. Shoulder Shrug

Stand erect with a slight arch in the lower back and a weight in each hand. The arms should be hanging at the sides of the body, with the elbows straight. Without bending the elbows, raise both shoulders as high as possible toward the ears; then pinch the shoulder blades back together (Fig. 39).

Each repetition involves the shoulders going up and then backwards, before returning to the starting position. Inhale as the shoulders are raised up and backwards, and exhale as the shoulders are lowered. This exercise is important for strengthening the upper back muscles and for reinforcing proper lifting posture.

3. Isometric Leg Raise

A properly performed isometric leg raise is a combination of the two following abdominal muscle functions: (1) stabilizing the pelvis in an upwardly rotated position to keep the lower back from arching and (2) compression of the abdominal cavity.

This exercise is important for strengthening the abdominal muscles used to (a) increase the intra-abdominal pressure when lifting, (b) support the intra-abdominal organs, and (c) maintain the proper alignment of the pelvis and lumbar spine in the erect standing position.

There are three progressions to this exercise: (1) single leg raise, (2) single leg raise with weight, and (3) double leg raise.

Before starting the leg raise exercises, however, one must get used to tightening isometrically the abdominal muscles used in lifting. Lie on the back with both knees bent and the feet flat on

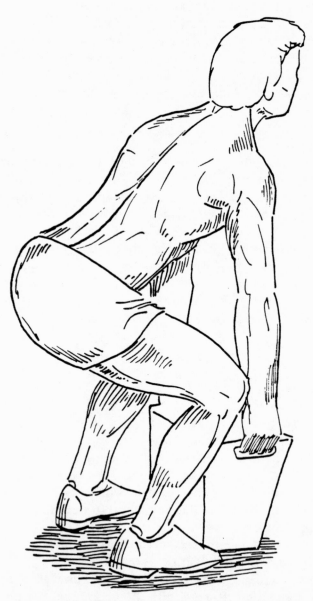

Figure 37. Proper starting position for lifting a low object from in front of the feet.

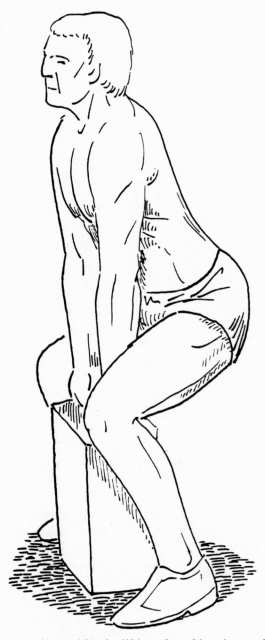

Figure 38. Proper starting position for lifting a low object that can be straddled.

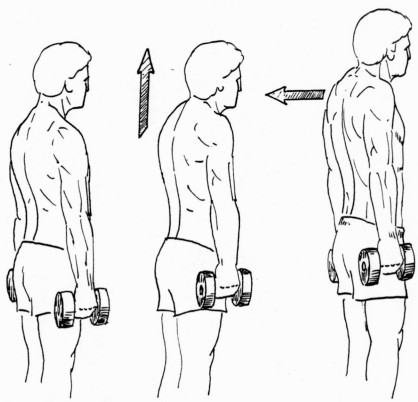

Figure 39. Shoulder shrug exercise. a. Starting position. b. Shoulders raised up. c. Shoulders moved backwards.

the floor (Fig. 40). Push your lower back flat against the floor by tightening up your abdominal muscles. Hold this position for two seconds and then relax. It is natural to hold one's breath slightly during this exercise, as it is during all of the leg raise progressions. When this exercise has been easily mastered with knees bent for ten repetitions, progress to the same exercise with the knees just slightly bent (Fig. 41). One can start the isometric leg raise progression when this exercise has been easily mastered for ten repetitions with the knees slightly bent.

In all the leg raise progressions, the lower back must not be allowed to arch.[45] It must be kept flat against the floor during the leg raise. Otherwise, the abdominal muscles will not be worked

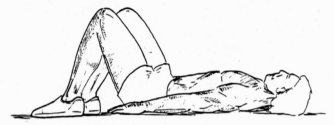

Figure 40. Supine position with both knees bent for isometrically tightening the abdominal muscles.

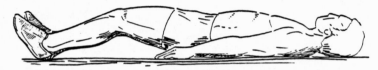

Figure 41. Supine position with the knees just slightly bent for isometrically tightening the abdominal muscles.

properly. In each progression, the heel is held about six inches (15 cm) off the floor for two seconds. This is one repetition.

1. Single Leg Raise

For the single leg raise (Fig. 42), keep one heel on the floor with the knee slightly bent. Keep the hands at the sides of the body.

Tighten the abdominal muscles so the lower back is kept flat against the floor. Then, raise the other leg, keeping the knee slightly bent, until the heel is about 6 inches off the floor. Hold this position for two seconds. Then, lower the leg and exhale.

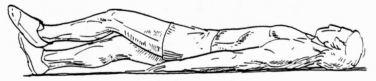

Figure 42. Single leg raise.

2. Single Leg Raise With Weight

When the single leg raise can be done easily for ten repetitions, place a one pound (0.5 kg) weight across the front of the ankle. The single leg raise is performed exactly the same way with weights (Fig. 43). Be sure to keep the knee slightly bent on the leg holding the weight off the floor. Bend the knee even more when lowering the leg back to the floor, to avoid stressing the lower back.

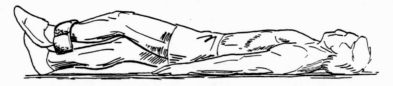

Figure 43. Single leg raise with a weight across the ankle.

3. Double Leg Raise

After doing single leg raises with weights for several months, attempt a double leg raise. Keeping the lower back flat against the floor, raise both heels six inches off the floor while keeping the knees fully flexed (Fig. 44). Hold this position for two seconds. (It may be easier to stabilize one's upper trunk during this exercise by keeping the arms above the head, holding onto the legs of a chair. This will be necessary for individuals with heavy legs, or with long legs compared to the length of the trunk.)

If the double leg raise with fully flexed knees can be done without arching the lower back, progress to this exercise. Be sure only to raise the heels about six inches off the floor, and hold each repetition for only two seconds.

After ten repetitions can be performed in the double leg raise with full knee flexion, progress to a double leg raise with less knee bend. As the abdominal muscles strengthen, do the double leg raise with less and less knee bend.

The final progression is the double leg raise with the knees just

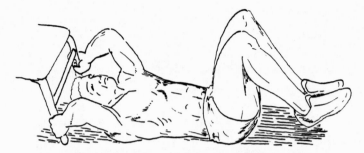

Figure 44. Double leg raise with both knees bent.

slightly bent (Fig. 45). Having the knees slightly bent as opposed to fully extended will make it easier to keep the lower back from arching. However, be sure to bend both knees fully when lowering the legs back to the floor after each repetition, to avoid stressing the lower back.

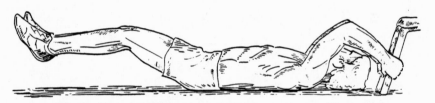

Figure 45. Double leg raise with the knees just slightly bent.

Eventually, work up to ten repetitions in the double leg raise with slightly bent knees. However, do not rush into doing this exercise. The double leg raise with slightly bent knees will be extremely difficult for most adolescents and adults to perform without arching their lower backs, which is to be absolutely avoided (Fig. 46).

EXERCISE SCHEDULE

The leg stretches and back extension exercise can be done every day. It is especially important to do these exercises immediately before any planned heavy lifting activities are attempted. The

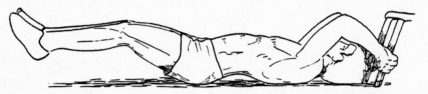

Figure 46. Incorrect double leg raise technique. Note the arch in the lower back.

back extension exercise is critical if prior to any lifting, one has been sitting for a prolonged period of time in a flexed posture.[1]

The resistive exercises should only be done three times a week, on alternate days, and not two days in a row.

Chapter 5

PROPER SITTING POSTURE
AND EXERCISE APPLICATIONS

The proper way to sit is with the normal lordosis present in the erect standing position (Fig. 47). Prolonged sitting with a flat or flexed lower back, as opposed to a lordotic posture, will stretch the posterior fibrous wall of the discs and posterior ligaments of the back, as well as cause a greater pressure increase within the discs.[4,5,44,54]

REASONS FOR IMPROPER SITTING POSTURE

There are many reasons why an individual, even after proper instruction, cannot sit properly. Some of these reasons are from muscle tightness and a lack of mobility. The other reasons relate to poorly designed chairs.

Muscle Tightness and Lack of Mobility

Tight Hamstrings

The hamstring muscles, when tight, will keep the lumbar spine flexed when sitting by rotating the pelvis upward (Fig. 48). Many people have difficulty keeping a normal lordosis in the lower back when sitting with their knees straight due to excessive hamstring tension.

With extremely tight hamstrings, it will even be difficult to keep a normal lordosis with the knees bent.[90] This is one important reason for proper hamstring stretching (see Chapter 4).

53

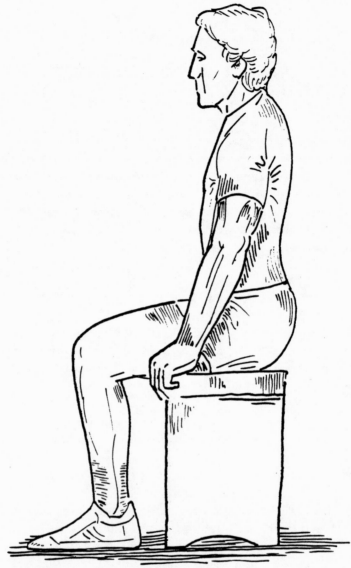

Figure 47. Proper sitting posture with lumbar lordosis.

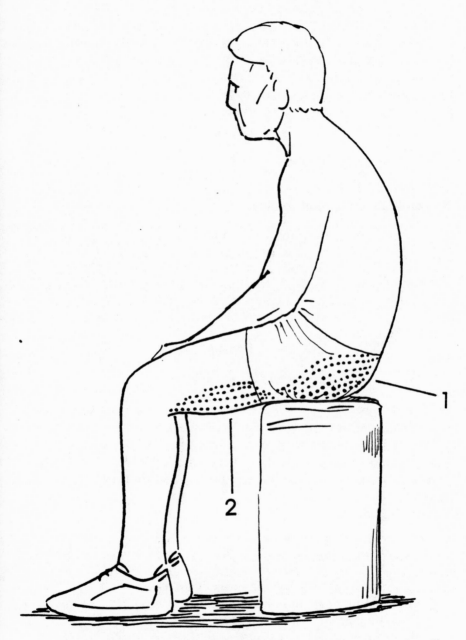

Figure 48. When sitting, tight hamstring (2) and gluteus maximus (1) muscles will force the lower back to flex due to their pull on the pelvis.

Tight Gluteus Maximus

When tight, gluteus maximus muscles can also contribute to flexing the lumbar spine when sitting by rotating the pelvis upward (Fig. 48). Leg stretching exercise number three in Chapter 4 is important to stretch this muscle.

One reason individuals often move their buttocks forward in upright chairs is to reduce the tension in their hamstrings and gluteus maximus muscles that is causing excessive flexion of the lower back (Fig. 49).[44]

Loss of Back Extension Mobility

As a result of keeping the lumbar spine flexed day after day, some individuals may have lost the ability to extend their lumbar spine sufficiently.[63] Therefore, they are not able to obtain a normal lordosis when sitting. For these individuals, the standing back extension exercise is important (see Chapter 4).

Poorly Designed Chairs

Thigh to Trunk Angle at 90 Degrees or Less

The lumbar spine will be forced into flexion very easily when the angle between an individual's thigh and trunk is 90 degrees or less.[30] This may be due to the angle between the chair seat and backrest being at 90 degrees or less (Fig. 50), from too soft a seat, or from the seat being too low to the floor so the knees are much higher than the hips (Fig. 51). The latter is often a problem with tall individuals.

No Lower Back Support

Chairs that do not have a support for the lower back to help maintain the normal lumbar lordosis are poorly designed. A proper lumbar support will reduce the disc pressure and muscle activity in the lower back by preventing the lumbar spine from flexing (Fig. 52).[3,5]

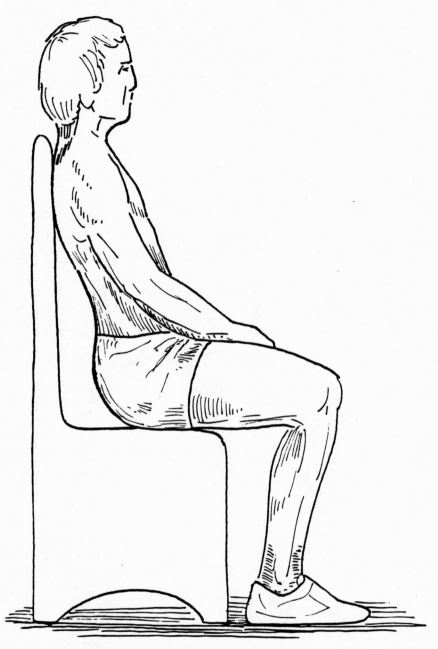

Figure 49. Moving the buttocks forward on the chair seat, to reduce the tension in the hamstring and gluteus maximus muscles.

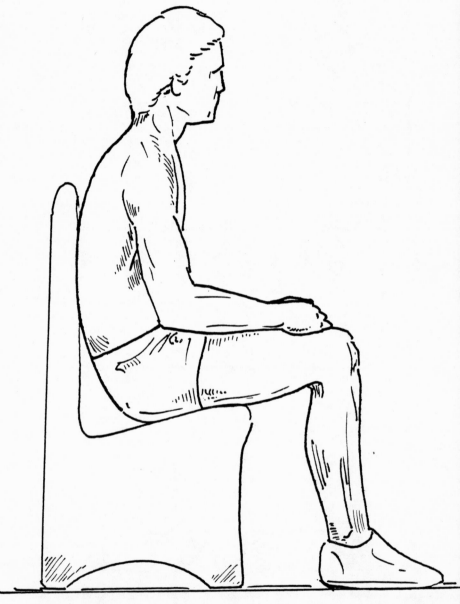

Figure 50. Example of a poorly designed chair. The angle between the chair seat and backrest is less than 90 degrees.

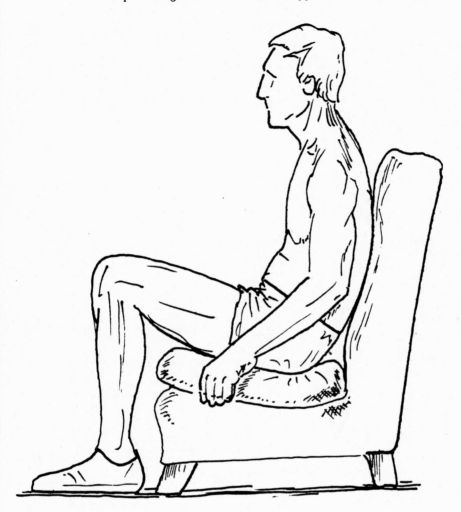

Figure 51. Example of a seat too low to the floor, resulting in excessive flexion of the lumbar spine.

Lumbar supports are available commercially that can be attached to any chair or car seat.

Excessive Seat Depth

With excessive seat depth, the individual will scoot forward on the seat, in order to remove pressure from behind the knees (Fig.

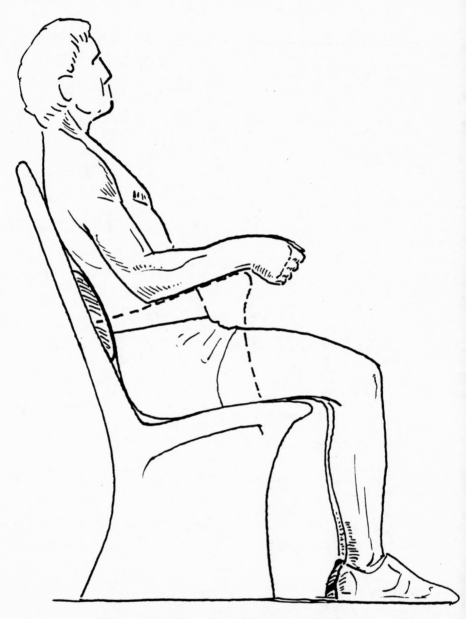

Figure 52. Proper lumbar support for the lower back.

53). Therefore, the individual will not sit properly against the backrest but will slouch. Even if a lumbar support was present on the chair, one would not be able to use it properly.

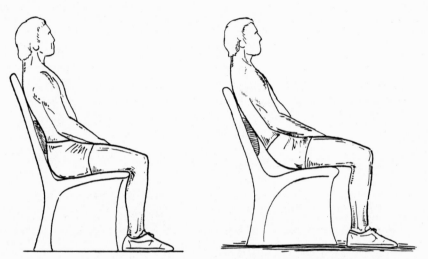

Figure 53. a. Excessive seat depth, resulting in pressure behind the knees. b. Slouched posture adapted in order to remove pressure from behind the knees.

Back Upholstery Too Soft

In this instance, due to a lack of proper support, the lumbar spine will easily assume a flexed position.

Vertical Backrest

There will be a greater potential for muscle fatigue in the lower back and a greater disc pressure with a vertical backrest, compared to having the backrest slightly inclined.[5]

Chairs without Armrests

In chairs without armrests, there will be an increase in muscle activity from the trapezius muscles (Fig. 54).[5] The increased trapezius muscle activity is necessary in order to support the free-hanging arms. Upper back and neck pain will often result from this posture.

Chairs without Backrests (Stools, Bleachers)

Individuals must be taught to actively contract the lower back muscles to keep the normal lumbar lordosis on these seats (Fig. 55). Strong back muscles, strengthened properly as stabilizers of the lumbar spine, are therefore important. Due to muscle fatigue, however, this posture cannot be held for prolonged time periods.

Lack of an Inclined Desk Surface

Even with the proper lumbar support and backrest, the individual will not be able to make use of them if he has to flex forward over a horizontal desk surface (Fig. 56). The use of an inclined desk surface will result in a less stressful position for the lower back, upper back, and neck (Fig. 57).[22]

PROPER CHAIR DESIGN

For prolonged sitting, a good chair should have the following features (see Figs. 52 and 57):[21, 35, 84, 104]

A. Seat to backrest angles from 95 to 105 degrees.
B. Lower back support.
C. A seat height that allows the feet to rest comfortably on the floor. Excessive pressure under the thighs can interfere with the venous blood flow from the legs.[69, 80]
D. A seat depth that avoids pressure behind the knee.
E. An inclined backrest that provides scapular support.
F. An inclined seat to help keep one's back against the backrest and lumbar support, and prevent sliding forward on the seat.
G. Seat and back upholstery that are not soft, but moderately firm. A hard seat will be more comfortable with a slight

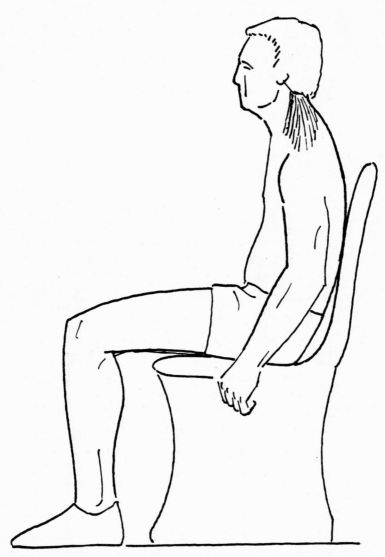

Figure 54. Increase in trapezius muscle activity (shaded area) from sitting in a chair without armrests.

contouring for the buttocks. The seat cover should not be slippery, as this will facilitate sliding forward on the seat.

H. Armrests that properly support the weight of the arms.

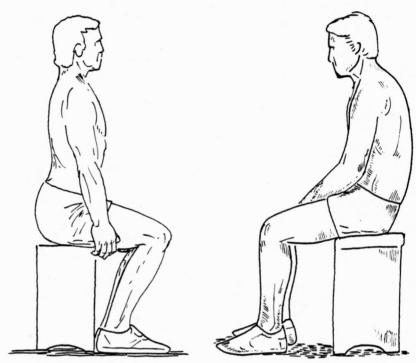

Figure 55. a. Proper sitting posture in a chair without a backrest. b. Incorrect sitting posture in a chair without a backrest.

When the armrests are too high, they will elevate the shoulders and cause discomfort. If the armrests are too low, the individual will slouch or lean to one side for some arm support.[21]

I. An inclined desk surface.

An inclined seat, inclined backrest, and lumbar support are also critical to provide proper sitting stability and comfort in cars, trucks, and wheelchairs. The improved posture and pressure distribution with these features will help reduce the spinal trauma from vibration and road shock.[94]

For prolonged alert sitting postures (reading, writing, lectures, conversation, driving), a backrest inclination of 15 to 20 degrees from vertical is recommended.[21,35,84,94,104] A headrest will be necessary on easy chairs with a backrest inclination greater than 30 degrees from vertical.[21]

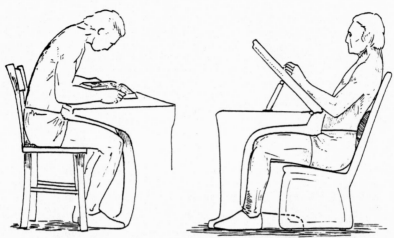

Figure 56. Spinal flexion that occurs when using a horizontal desk.

Figure 57. Inclining the desk surface will reduce the stress on the spine.

Chapter 6

POTENTIALLY HARMFUL EXERCISES

FLEXION

Any exercises that involve forceful flexion, or a combination of flexion–lateral bending or flexion rotation should be avoided due to the potentially harmful stress put on the discs and posterior ligaments of the lower back. These exercises also reinforce the movement pattern of spinal flexion with hip flexion, which will contribute to ingraining poor lifting technique in many individuals. Examples of such exercises include the following toe touching movements:

A. Toe touches standing with the knees straight (Fig. 58).
B. Alternate toe touches standing with the knees straight (Fig. 59).
C. Toe touches sitting with the knees straight (Fig. 60).
D. Alternate toe touches, sitting with the knees straight (Fig. 61).

These exercises are a poor test of hamstring flexibility.[49] The ability to touch one's toes with the knees straight can vary, depending on one's body proportions. Toe touching can also be accomplished by individuals with tight hamstrings who have an overstretched lower back. By attempting to forcefully touch one's toes with tight hamstrings and straight knees, one can harmfully overstress the lower back.

For stretching the hamstrings, the hamstring stretch with rope (*see* Chapter 4) is superior to the above exercises because it avoids putting a harmful stretch on the posterior aspect of the discs and posterior ligaments of the lower back. By holding one leg firmly against the floor, spinal flexion is minimized.

For back mobility in flexion, a supine flexion exercise (Fig. 62)

66

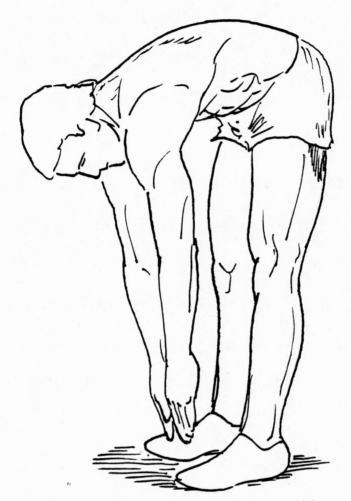

Figure 58. Toe touches standing with the knees straight.

will maintain the range of motion of the lower back in flexion, without any excessive stretching. For this exercise, one should lie on the back with both knees bent and the feet flat on the floor. Using the abdominal and hip flexor muscles, slowly bring both legs toward the chest until the lower back is just flattened, without forcing this movement. Then, lower the legs to the starting position.

The following sit-up exercises may also be potentially harmful:

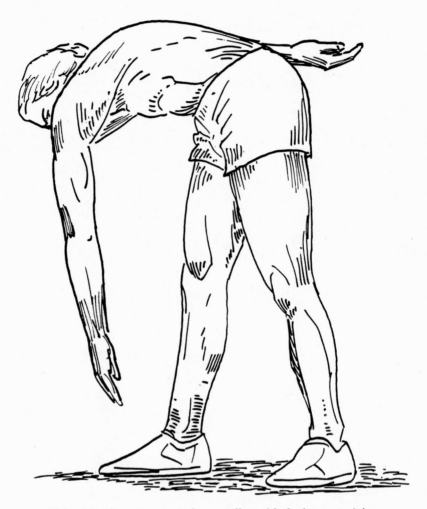

Figure 59. Alternate toe touches standing with the knees straight.

A. Full sit-ups with bent knees (Fig. 63).
B. Full sit-ups with straight knees (Fig. 64).
C. Full sit-ups with trunk rotation (Fig. 65).

Full sit-ups should be avoided due to the excessive flexion of the lower back and great increase in disc pressure that results from

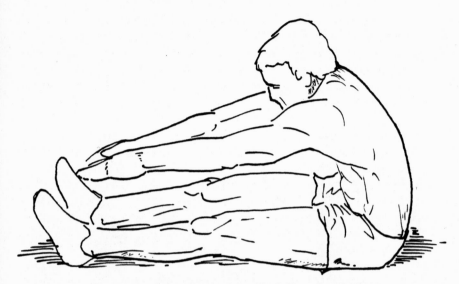

Figure 60. Toe touches sitting with the knees straight.

this exercise. Full sit-ups have been mentioned by other authors as possibly contributing to disc degeneration.[37,101]

Sit-ups with the knees straight will cause more stress to the lower back than bent knee sit-ups due to the excessive tension in the hamstrings that will limit one's hip mobility.

If one prefers to do sit-up exercises, a partial sit-up done with the knees bent, and only elevating the head and shoulder blades off the floor, is the safest technique (Fig. 66).

Weight lifting exercises in spinal flexion should be avoided, such as the following:

A. Bent over rowing (Fig. 67)
B. Deadlifts with the knees straight (Fig. 68)[67]
C. Bent over twists (Fig. 69)

The use of weights in these flexed positions will increase the stress on the lower back even more. Deadlifts should always be done with the hips and knees bent, keeping the lower back slightly arched (Fig. 70).

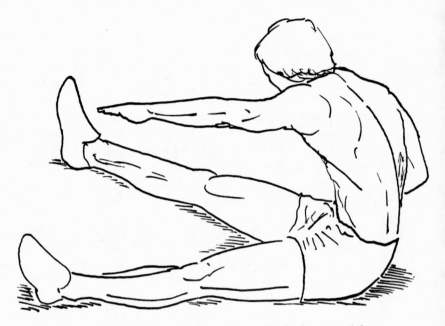

Figure 61. Alternate toe touches sitting with the knees straight.

FORCEFUL HYPEREXTENSION

Weight lifting exercises that result in repetitive, forceful hyper-extension (extreme backward bending) should also be avoided, such as overhead presses with extreme back arching (Fig. 71).[67,93] The repetitive trauma from these movements may eventually result in a stress fracture of the lower lumbar vertebrae (spondylolysis).[40,55]

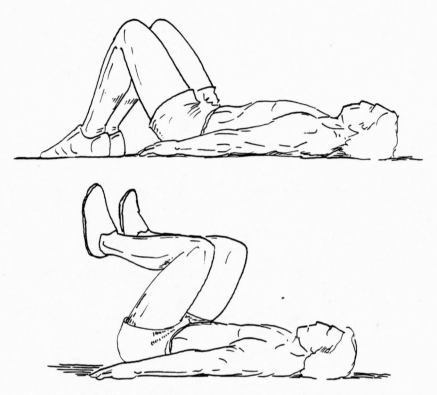

Figure 62. Supine flexion exercise for the lower back. a. Starting position. b. Top position. Both legs are brought towards the chest until the lower back just flattens.

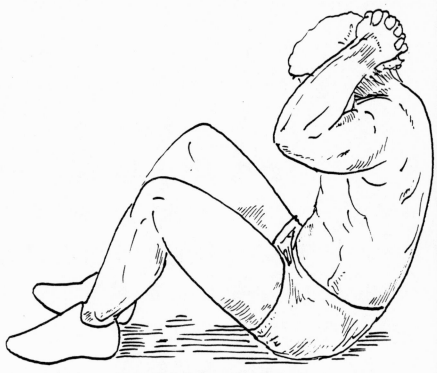

Figure 63. Full sit-up with bent knees.

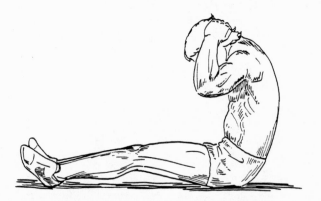

Figure 64. Full sit-up with straight knees.

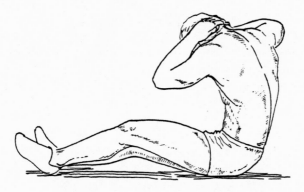

Figure 65. Full sit-up with trunk rotation.

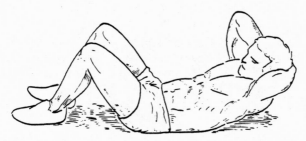

Figure 66. Partial sit-up, only elevating the head and shoulder blades off the floor.

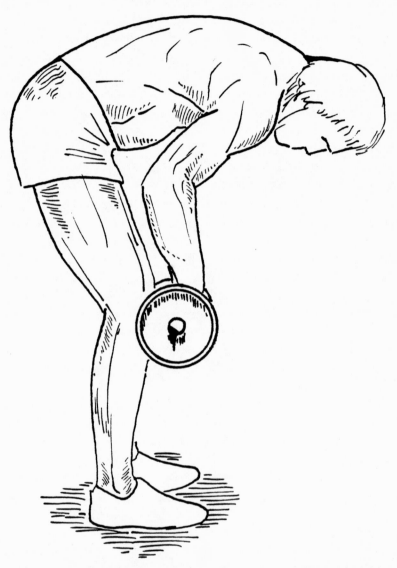

Figure 67. Bent over rowing exercise. While staying in a bent forward position, the individual brings the barbell up to the chest or abdomen by bending the elbows.

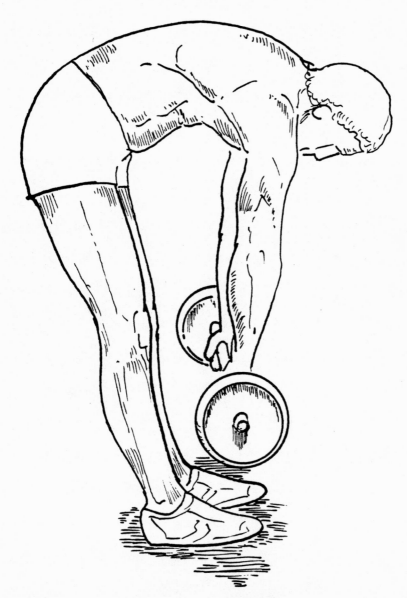

Figure 68. Deadlifts with the knees straight. Keeping the knees straight, the individual bends over and touches the barbell to the floor. The individual then returns to the erect standing position without bending the knees.

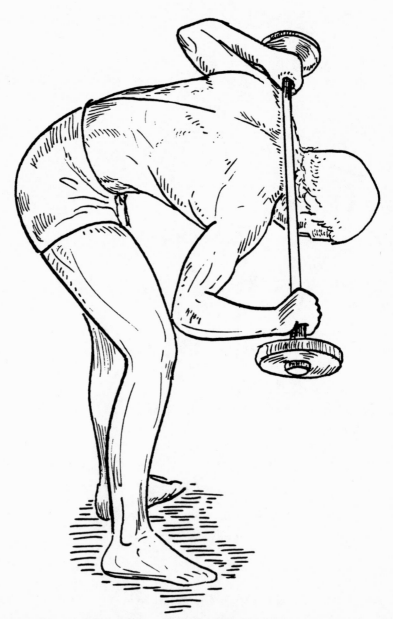

Figure 69. Bent over twists. While staying in the bent forward position, the individual rotates the barbell and trunk from side to side.

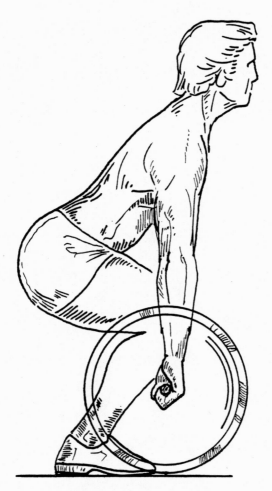

Figure 70. Proper deadlift technique. The lower back muscles are tightened to keep the lumbar spine in a slightly arched position. The hips and knees are bent, and the head is kept up.

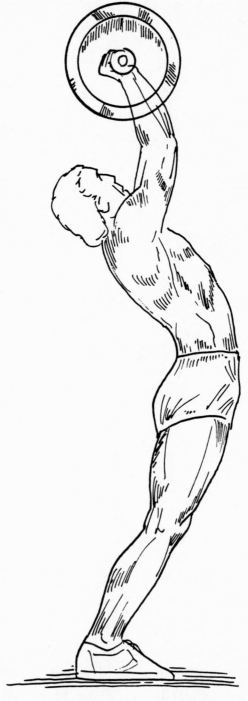

Figure 71. Overhead press with extreme back arching.

REFERENCES

1. Adams, M. A., and Hutton, W. C.: Prolapsed intervertebral disc. A hyper-flexion injury. *Spine, 7*:184–191, 1982.
2. Adams, M. A., and Hutton, W. C.: The effect of fatigue on the lumbar intervertebral disc. *The Journal of Bone and Joint Surgery, 65–B*:199–203, 1983.
3. Åkerblom, B.: *Standing and Sitting Posture*. Stockholm, Nordiska Bokhandeln, 1948.
4. Andersson, B. J. G., Örtengren, R., Nachemson, A., and Elfström, G.: Lumbar disc pressure and myoelectric back muscle activity during sitting. 1. Studies on an experimental chair. *Scandinavian Journal of Rehabilitation Medicine, 6*:104–114, 1974.
5. Andersson, B. J. G., Örtengren, R., Nachemson, A. L., Elfström, G., and Broman, H.: The sitting posture: an electromyographic and discometric study. *Orthopedic Clinics of North America, 6*:105–120, 1975.
6. Andersson, G. B. J., Örtengren, R., and Nachemson, A.: Quantitative studies of back loads in lifting. *Spine, 1*:178–185, 1976.
7. Ariel, B. G.: Biomechanical analysis of the knee joint during deep knee bends with heavy load. In Nelson, R. C., and Morehouse, C. A. (Eds.): *Biomechanics IV. International Series on Sport Sciences*. Baltimore, Univ Park, 1974, vol. 1, pp. 44–52.
8. Asmussen, E., and Klausen, K.: Form and function of the erect human spine. *Clinical Orthopaedics, 25*:55–63, 1962.
9. Bartelink, D. L.: The role of abdominal pressure in relieving the pressure on the lumbar intervertebral discs. *The Journal of Bone and Joint Surgery, 39–B*:718–725, 1957.
10. Basmajian, J. V.: *Muscles Alive. Their Functions Revealed by Electromyography*, 4th ed. Baltimore, Williams and Wilkins, 1978, p. 178.
11. Blackburn, S. E., and Portney, L. G.: Electromyographic activity of back musculature during Williams' flexion exercises. *Physical Therapy, 61*:878–885, 1981.
12. Boulton–Davies, I. M.: Physiotherapists—teachers of the public. *Physiotherapy, 65*:280, 1979.
13. Cady, L. D., Bischoff, D. P., O'Connell, E. R., Thomas, P. C., and Allan, J. H.: Authors' response. *Journal of Occupational Medicine, 21*:720, 725, 1979.

14. Chaffin, D. B., and Park, K. S.: A longitudinal study of low-back pain as associated with occupational weight lifting factors. *American Industrial Hygiene Association Journal, 34*:513–525, 1973.

15. Collins, G. A., Cohen, M. J., Naliboff, B. D., and Schandler, S. L.: Comparative analysis of paraspinal and frontalis EMG, heart rate and skin conductance in chronic low back pain patients and normals to various postures and stress. *Scandinavian Journal of Rehabilitation Medicine, 14*:39–46, 1982.

16. Cyriax, J.: *Textbook of Orthopaedic Medicine*, 7th ed. London, Bailliere Tindall, 1978, vol. 1.

17. Davis, P. R.: The causation of herniae by weight-lifting. *The Lancet, 2*:155–157, August 22, 1959.

18. Davis, P. R.: The physical causation of disease. *Royal Society of Health Journal, 92*:63–64, 1972.

19. Davis, P. R., and Troup, J. D. G.: Pressures in the trunk cavities when pulling, pushing and lifting. *Ergonomics, 7*:465–474, 1964.

20. Davis, P. R., Troup, J. D. G., and Burnard, J. H.: Movements of the thoracic and lumbar spine when lifting: a chrono-cyclophotographic study. *Journal of Anatomy, London, 99*:13–26, 1965.

21. Diffrient, N., Tilley, A. R., and Bardagjy, J. C.: *Humanscale 1/2/3.* Cambridge, MIT Pr, 1974.

22. Eastman, M. C., and Kamon, E.: Posture and subjective evaluation at flat and slanted desks. *Human Factors, 18*:15–25, 1976.

23. Edgar, M.: Pathologies associated with lifting. *Physiotherapy, 65*:245–247, 1979.

24. Eie, N.: Load capacity of the low back. *Journal of The Oslo City Hospitals, 16*:73–98, 1966.

25. Eie, N., and Wehn, P.: Measurements of the intra-abdominal pressure in relation to weight bearing of the lumbosacral spine. *Journal of The Oslo City Hospitals, 12*:205–217, 1962.

26. Ekholm, J., Arborelius, U. P., and Nemeth, G.: The load on the lumbosacral joint and trunk muscle activity during lifting. *Ergonomics, 25*:145–161, 1982.

27. Farfan, H. F.: *Mechanical Disorders of the Low Back.* Philadelphia, Lea and Febiger, 1973.

28. Farfan, H. F., Cossette, J. W., Robertson, G. H., Wells, R. V., and Kraus, H.: The effects of torsion on the lumbar intervertebral joints: the role of torsion in the production of disc degeneration. *The Journal of Bone and Joint Surgery, 52-A*:468–497, 1970.

29. Fisk, J. W.: *A Practical Guide to Management of The Painful Neck and Back. Diagnosis, Manipulation, Exercises, Prevention.* Springfield, Thomas, 1977.

30. Floyd, W. F., and Roberts, D. F.: Anatomical and physiological principles in chair and table design. *Ergonomics, 2*:1–16, 1958.

31. Floyd, W. F., and Silver, P. H. S.: Electromyographic study of patterns of

activity of the anterior abdominal wall muscles in man. *Journal of Anatomy,* *84*:132–145, 1950.

32. Floyd, W. F., and Silver, P. H. S.: The function of the erectores spinae muscles in certain movements and postures in man. *Journal of Physiology,* *129*:184–203, 1955.

33. Frymoyer, J. W., Pope, M. H., Clements, J. H., Wilder, D. G., MacPherson, B., and Ashikaga, T.: Risk factors in low-back pain. An epidemiological survey. *The Journal of Bone and Joint Surgery, 65-A*:213–218, 1983.

34. Garhammer, J.: Free weight equipment for the development of athletic strength and power — part 1. *National Strength and Conditioning Association Journal, 3*:24–26, 33, December 1981 – January 1982.

35. Grandjean, E., Hünting, W., Wotzka, G., and Schärer, R.: An ergonomic investigation of multipurpose chairs. *Human Factors, 15*:247–255, 1973.

36. Grillner, S., Nilsson, J., and Thorstensson, A.: Intra-abdominal pressure changes during natural movements in man. *Acta Physiologica Scandinavica, 103*:275–283, 1978.

37. Halpern, A. A., and Bleck, E. E.: Sit-up exercises: an electromyographic study. *Clinical Orthopaedics and Related Research, 145*:172–178, 1979.

38. Hickey, D. S., and Hukins, D. W. L.: Relation between the structure of the annulus fibrosus and the function and failure of the intervertebral disc. *Spine, 5*:106–116, 1980.

39. Inoue, H., and Takeda, T.: Three-dimensional observation of collagen framework of lumbar intervertebral discs. *Acta Orthopaedica Scandinavica, 46*:949–956, 1975.

40. Jackson, D. W., Wiltse, L. L., and Cirincione, R. J.: Spondylolysis in the female gymnast. *Clinical Orthopaedics and Related Research, 117*:68–73, 1976.

41. Jackson, J. M.: Biomechanical hazards in the dockworker. *Annals of Occupational Hygiene, 11*:147–157, 1968.

42. Jensen, G. M.: Biomechanics of the lumbar intervertebral disk: a review. *Physical Therapy, 60*:765–773, 1980.

43. Kapandji, I. A.: *The Physiology of the Joints,* 2nd ed. Edinburgh, Churchill, 1974, vol. 3.

44. Keegan, J. J.: Alterations of the lumbar curve related to posture and seating. *The Journal of Bone and Joint Surgery, 35-A*:589–603, 1953.

45. Kendall, F. P.: A criticism of current tests and exercises for physical fitness. *Journal of the American Physical Therapy Association, 45*:187–197, 626, 1965.

46. Kendall, H. O., and Kendall, F. P.: Normal flexibility according to age groups. *The Journal of Bone and Joint Surgery, 30-A*:690–694, 1948.

47. Kendall, H. O., Kendall, F. P., and Boynton, D. A.: *Posture and Pain.* Huntington, Krieger, 1970, p. 54.

48. King, A. I., Prasad, P., and Ewing, C. L.: Mechanism of spinal injury due to caudocephalad acceleration. *Orthopedic Clinics of North America, 6*:19–31, 1975.

49. Kisner, C.: Touching the toes. *The Physician and Sportsmedicine, 8*:18, March 1980.

50. Klausen, K., Nielsen, B., and Madsen, L.: Form and function of the spine in young males with and without "back troubles." In Morecki, A., Fidelus, K., Kedzior, K., and Wit, A. (Eds.): *Biomechanics VII-A. International Series on Biomechanics.* Baltimore, Univ Park, 1981, Vol. 3A, pp. 174–180.

51. Klein, J. A., Hickey, D. S., and Hukins, D. W. L.: Computer graphics illustration of the operation of the intervertebral disc. *Engineering in Medicine, 11*:11–15, 1982.

52. Klein, J. A., and Hukins, D. W. L.: Collagen fibre orientation in the annulus fibrosus of intervertebral disc during bending and torsion measured by x-ray diffraction. *Biochimica et Biophysica Acta, 719*:98–101, 1982.

53. Koreska, J., Gibson, D. A., and Albisser, A. M.: Structural support system for unstable spines. In Komi, P. V. (Ed.): *Biomechanics V-A. International Series on Biomechanics.* Baltimore, Univ Park, 1976, vol. 1-A, pp. 474–483.

54. Kottke, F. J.: Evaluation and treatment of low back pain due to mechanical causes. *Archives of Physical Medicine and Rehabilitation, 42*:426–440, 1961.

55. Kulund, D. N., Dewey, J. B., Brubaker, C. E., and Roberts, J. R.: Olympic weight-lifting injuries. *The Physician and Sportsmedicine, 6*:111–119, November 1978.

56. Kumar, S.: A study of spinal motion during lifting. *Irish Journal of Medical Science, 143*:86–95, 1974.

57. Kumar, S.: Physiological responses to weight lifting in different planes. *Ergonomics, 23*:987–993, 1980.

58. Kumar, S., and Davis, P. R.: Lumbar vertebral innervation and intra-abdominal pressure. *Journal of Anatomy, 114*:47–53, 1973.

59. Lin, H. S., Liu, Y. K., and Adams, K. H.: Mechanical response of the lumbar intervertebral joint under physiological (complex) loading. *The Journal of Bone and Joint Surgery, 60-A*:41–55, 1978.

60. Lindh, M.: Biomechanics of the lumbar spine. In Frankel, V. H., and Nordin, M. (Eds.): *Basic Biomechanics of the Skeletal System.* Philadelphia, Lea and Febiger, 1980, pp. 255–290.

61. Lipetz, S., and Gutin, B.: An electromyographic study of four abdominal exercises. *Medicine and Science in Sports, 2*:35–38, 1970.

62. Lorenz, M., Patwardhan, A., and Vanderby, R.: Load-bearing characteristics of lumbar facets in normal and surgically altered spinal segments. *Spine, 8*:122–130, 1983.

63. McKenzie, R. A.: *The Lumbar Spine. Mechanical Diagnosis and Therapy.* Waikanae, Spinal Publications, 1981.

64. Magora, A.: Investigation of the relation between low back pain and occupation. Three physical requirements: sitting, standing, and weight lifting. *Industrial Medicine, 41*:5–9, December 1972.

65. Magora, A.: Investigation of the relation between low back pain and occupation. IV. Physical requirements: bending, rotation, reaching and

sudden maximal effort. *Scandinavian Journal of Rehabilitation Medicine*, 5:186–190, 1973.

66. Markolf, K. L., and Morris, J. M.: The structural components of the intervertebral disc. A study of their contributions to the ability of the disc to withstand compressive forces. *The Journal of Bone and Joint Surgery*, 56-A:675–687, 1974.

67. Mason, T. A.: Is weight lifting deleterious to the spines of young people? *British Journal of Sports Medicine*, 5:54–56, July 1970.

68. Miles, M., and Sullivan, W. E.: Lateral bending at the lumbar and lumbosacral joints. *The Anatomical Record*, 139:387–393, 1961.

69. Morimoto, S.: Effect of sitting posture on human body. *The Bulletin of Tokyo Medical and Dental University*, 20:19–34, 1973.

70. Morris, J. M.: Intervertebral disc disease of the lumbosacral spine: biomechanical and clinical observations. In Brown, F. W. (Ed.): *Symposium on The Lumbar Spine*. St. Louis, Mosby, 1981, pp. 3–15.

71. Mundale, M. O., Hislop, H. J., Rabideau, R. J., and Kottke, F. J.: Evaluation of extension of the hip. *Archives of Physical Medicine and Rehabilitation*, 37:75–80, 1956.

72. Nachemson, A.: The load on lumbar disks in different positions of the body. *Clinical Orthopedics*, 45:107–122, 1966.

73. Nachemson, A.: Towards a better understanding of low-back pain: a review of the mechanics of the lumbar disc. *Rheumatology and Rehabilitation*, 14:129–143, 1975.

74. Nachemson, A. L.: Low back pain. Its etiology and treatment. *Clinical Medicine*, 78:18–24, 1971.

75. Nachemson, A. L.: The lumbar spine. An orthopaedic challenge. *Spine*, 1:59–71, 1976.

76. Nachemson, A., and Elfström, G.: Intravital dynamic pressure measurements in lumbar discs. A study of common movements, maneuvers and exercises. *Scandinavian Journal of Rehabilitation Medicine, Supplement 1*:1–40, 1970.

77. Nachemson, A. L., Schultz, A. B., and Berkson, M. H.: Mechanical properties of human lumbar spine motion segments. Influences of age, sex, disc level, and degeneration. *Spine*, 4:1–8, 1979.

78. Newman, P. H.: Sprung back. *The Journal of Bone and Joint Surgery*, 34-b:30–37, 1952.

79. Ono, K.: Electromyographic studies of the abdominal wall muscles in visceroptosis. 1. Analysis of patterns of activity of the abdominal wall muscles in normal adults. *The Tohoku Journal of Experimental Medicine*, 68:347–354, 1958.

80. Pottier, M., Dubreuil, A., and Monod, H.: The effects of sitting posture on the volume of the foot. *Ergonomics*, 12:753–758, 1969.

81. Poulsen, E.: Back muscle strength and weight limits in lifting burdens. *Spine*, 6:73–75, 1981.

82. Rab, G. T., Chao, E. Y. S., and Stauffer, R. N.: Muscle force analysis of the lumbar spine. *Orthopedic Clinics of North America,* 8:193–199, 1977.

83. Rasch, P. J., and Burke, R. K.: *Kinesiology and Applied Anatomy. The Science of Human Movement,* 6th ed. Philadelphia, Lea and Febiger, 1978, pp. 242–243.

84. Ridder, C. A.: *Basic Design Measurements For Sitting.* Bulletin 616, Agricultural Experiment Station, University of Arkansas, Fayetteville, October 1959.

85. Sale, D., and MacDougall, D.: Specificity in strength training: a review for the coach and athlete. *Canadian Journal of Applied Sport Sciences,* 6:87–92, 1981.

86. Shah, J. S., Hampson, W. G. J., and Jayson, M. I. V.: The distribution of surface strain in the cadaveric lumbar spine. *The Journal of Bone and Joint Surgery, 60-B:*246–251, 1978.

87. Snook, S. H., Campanelli, R. A., and Hart, J. W.: A study of three preventive approaches to low back injury. *Journal of Occupational Medicine, 20:*478–481, 1978.

88. Soderberg, G. L., and Barr, J. O.: Muscular function in chronic low back dysfunction. *Spine, 8:*79–85, 1983.

89. Stillwell, G. K.: The Law of Laplace. Some clinical applications. *Mayo Clinic Proceedings, 48:*863–869, 1973.

90. Stokes, I. A. F., and Abery, J. M.: Influence of the hamstring muscles on lumbar spine curvature in sitting. *Spine, 5:*525–528, 1980.

91. Strachan, A.: Back care in industry. *Physiotherapy, 65:*249–251, 1979.

92. Troup, J. D. G.: Relation of lumbar spine disorders to heavy manual work and lifting. *The Lancet, 1:*857–861, April 17, 1965.

93. Troup, J. D. G.: The risk of weight-training and weight-lifting in young people. *British Journal of Sports Medicine, 5:*27–33, July 1970.

94. Troup, J. D. G.: Driver's back pain and its prevention. *Applied Ergonomics,* 9:207–214, 1978.

95. Troup, J. D. G., and Chapman, A. E.: The strength of the flexor and extensor muscles of the trunk. *Journal of Biomechanics, 2:*49–62, 1969.

96. Vrijens, J.: Muscle strength development in the pre- and post-pubescent age. *Medicine and Sport, 11:*152–158, 1978.

97. Watanabe, K.: Biomechanical implications of EMG activity of erector spinae and gluteus maximus muscles in postural changes of the trunk. In Morecki, A., Fidelus, K., Kedzior, K., and Wit, A. (Eds.): *Biomechanics VII-B. International Series on Biomechanics.* Baltimore, Univ Park, 1981, Vol. 3B, pp. 23–30.

98. Weltman, A., and Stamford, B.: Strength training: free weights vs. machines. *The Physician and Sportsmedicine, 10:*197, November 1982.

99. White, A. A., and Gordon, S. L.: Synopsis: workshop on idiopathic low-back pain. *Spine, 7:*141–149, 1982.

100. White, A. A., and Panjabi, M. M.: *Clinical Biomechanics of the Spine.* Philadelphia, Lippincott, 1978, p. 285.

101. White, A. A., and Panjabi, M. M.: *Clinical Biomechanics of the Spine*. Philadelphia, Lippincott, 1978, p. 306.
102. Wiles, P.: Postural deformities of the anteroposterior curves of the spine. *The Lancet, 1*:911–919, April 17, 1937.
103. Wolf, S. L., Basmajian, J. V., Russe, C. T. C., and Kutner, M.: Normative data on low back mobility and activity levels. *American Journal of Physical Medicine, 58*:217–229, 1979.
104. Wotzka, G., Grandjean, E., Burandt, U., Kretzschmar, H., and Leonhard, T.: Investigations for the development of an auditorium seat. In Grandjean, E. (Ed.): *Sitting Posture*. London, Taylor and Francis, 1969, pp. 68–83.
105. Wyke, B.: The neurology of low back pain. In Jayson, M. I. V. (Ed.): *The Lumbar Spine and Back Pain*, 2nd ed. Tunbridge Wells, Pitman Medical, 1980, p. 266.

INDEX